Disclaimer

The material in this book is intended for information only. None of the suggestions are meant in any way to be prescriptive. Any attempt to treat a medical condition should always come under the direction of a competent physician and neither I or the publisher can accept responsibility for injuries or illness arising out of the failure of the reader to take medical advice.

This book is for informational purposes only. As each individual situation is unique, you should use proper discretion, discuss your condition with a health care practitioner, before undertaking any of the techniques or treatments described in this book. The author and publisher expressly disclaim responsibility for any adverse effects that may result from the use or application of the information contained in this book.

I want to make it clear that I have no commercial interest in any product, treatment or organization mentioned in this book.

Contents

1. My story - Why write this book?

2. What to do if you have a cold sore now

3. The life cycle of a cold sore

4. Products I have tried

5. Knowing your vulnerability

6. The perfect storm - The outbreak

7. Dealing with an outbreak

8. Stopping cold sores for good - Conclusion

Appendix A - Lysine - Arginine Tables

1.   My story - Why write this book?

Many years ago I had a blister develop on my lip. At first, I thought it was a pimple, but soon I began to realize this was no ordinary spot. It grew....and grew....and then blistered and scabbed. I didn't even know what it was. I just figured it was a one time event. But then a few weeks later the same thing happened and after another occurrence and some searching on the internet, I realized I was getting cold sores.

With the next outbreak, I went to the doctor. I found the whole thing was getting me down. I didn't want to go out or see friends and I was horrified to learn that I had contracted the Herpes Simplex Virus Type 1 (HSV1). I remember the doctor saying there wasn't a cure and it was *no big deal* and prescribing some antiviral drugs that would help clear it up.

No big deal. It certainly was a big deal to me. I felt like asking the doctor to stick a penny piece to his lip and to walk around for a few days and see how he felt. I sensed people were staring at my lip. I felt very self conscious and every time I got a cold sore, it would take two weeks out of my life. I would cancel all engagements and live like a hermit. I dreaded telling a new girlfriend. In fairness friends and family love you regardless, but when your self esteem is so low you want even the people who are dear to you to empathize. They would be kind and say it wasn't that noticeable. Telling them the feeling of a penny piece on your lip was a good way to help them understand how you felt.

After I while I resolved that I was going to find a way to stop getting cold sores. I spent countless hours on the internet, bought all the books I could find and tried several miracle cures. Over a period of several years I have established what works and what doesn't. Lots doesn't!

Having gone from several outbreaks a year, I have now reached a point where I can go over a year without getting a cold sore. On the rare occasion that I do get one, I know what caused the outbreak and kick myself for being so stupid. More importantly, I can stop the cold sore dead in its tracks so people don't notice it and have it cleared up in a day or two rather than a week or two.

This book is not a miracle cure. It offers practical advice on how to stop getting cold sores and what to do if all else fails and you find yourself having to deal with one that has slipped through the net. So why write this book? It is the book I wished I had available to me years ago. It would have saved me quite a bit of heartache and a lot of time searching for the answers. It would also have saved me quite a bit of money too, on other books and treatments that didn't work. Most of all, it would have saved me cancelling quite a lot of business meetings and dates. Who knows the cost of that?

But my real motivation for writing this book, is to share my own findings so you too can dramatically reduce the impact of getting cold sores in your life. Be patient. use this book as a reference each time you get a cold sore. I hope you learn what works for you and I hope it helps you.

Second Edition Update – Christmas 2019

Four years ago I wrote this book partly to record everything I had learned about living with and dealing with cold sores. I have found it to be a useful reference and refresher for myself. But in referring to it recently, I have realized I have discovered quite a few things since the first edition which I needed to share with you.

The first of the three main areas I have expanded on is the use of ice to dramatically reduce the scale and time of an outbreak. Indeed used early enough it is possible to reverse a cold sore altogether. I have use the market leading Zovirax cream more in recent years but in a particular way at a particular time which I have explained more fully. Last of all I have found raising my overall nutrition level by making soups with a soup maker has increased my overall immunity such that I rarely get the onslaught of a cold sore now, maybe one a year on average. And when this does happen, I can stop it in its tracks in a day or two. I really hope this book will help you to do the same.

I welcome any feedback at: coldsorebook@gmail.com

I am also very grateful for a review, no matter how short, on Amazon

2.   What to do if you have a cold sore now

This book is designed to help you understand how to stop getting cold sores and prevent outbreaks on an ongoing basis, but the chances are you are reading it because you have one right now and you want it to go away. Like yesterday!

So, if you hove a cold sore now that:

a) is coming, but not yet blistered (i.e. skin hasn't burst)

If you are fortunate enough to know you have one coming (although you don't feel very fortunate the moment you realize this). We can probably stop it. Great if you can get to a pharmacy. You will need to buy three or four basic off the shelf products. Next time we will be more prepared. But don't worry if you can't get to a pharmacy, we can still probably stop it in its tracks. **Go to the start of chapter 7, Dealing with an outbreak.**

If you think you have one coming but are not sure look up *Tingling* in the next chapter.

b) has blistered and burst

Now you need to minimize the risk of infection and passing the virus on to others. We also need to prevent the forming of a scab or reduce its size. **Go to the start of chapter 7, Dealing with an outbreak and read from 'Early treatment'.**

c) has a scab forming

We are now focused on reducing and the length of time you have the scab for and ensuring you have no scarring. **Go to the start of chapter 7, Dealing with an outbreak and read from 'If you have a scab forming.'**

BUT, before you go straight to these pages, please remember this book is mostly about how to stop getting a cold sore in the first place. If you have one, you need to deal with it now, but don't then just deal with your current situation and put this book down until the next time you have one. In the case of cold sores, ***prevention is much better than cure!***

3.   The life cycle of a cold sore

A cold sore is a fluid-filled blister that normally forms at the edge of a person's lips. The blisters often group together in very small patches. After the blisters break a scab forms over the sore. They usually take a couple of weeks to heal without leaving a scar. They are caused by the herpes simplex virus (HSV-1) which is contracted by close contact with another person with a cold sore, usually kissing.

There is no cure for HSV infection. Cold sore outbreaks may reoccur frequently depending on a variety of factors covered in this book. The most common form of medical treatment is with antiviral drugs, but this book explores preventing outbreaks and stopping cold sores fully developing. The most common reasons given for the cause of an outbreak are:

- having another infection
- having a high temperature, fever
- emotional upset or psychological stress
- tiredness and fatigue
- an injury to the infected area
- menstruation (periods)
- strong sunlight

There are some more causes and many triggers for an outbreak which we will look at further in chapter 5.

It is worth understanding the phases of an outbreak. I have broken this down into many more phases than you would normally read about because it is important to understand the whole process end to end.

1. Contraction

This is when you are first exposed to HSV-1. It is most likely from kissing someone else who is in the phases of an outbreak. It could be from a contaminated glass, shared water bottle, towel etc. It is quite likely that you will not know you have contracted the virus until your first (maybe even your second) outbreak. Once you have the virus, your own awareness and hygiene is vital in order not to pass it on to family or friends.

2. Virus laying dormant

HSV-1 lives in facial nerve cells and lies dormant until it senses a vulnerability or gateway to emerge as sore. The early outbreaks after contracting HSV1 are typically the worst and may be more frequent in the first year. After a while you can get better and better at reducing outbreaks or stopping them all together. But you need to be aware that the virus is always sitting there waiting for an opportunity to catch you off guard and break out.

3. Susceptibility

This is an aspect that is hardly written about and therefore forms a big part of this book. If you have a cold sore outbreak it is almost certainly because your immune system was at a low ebb. This can be for a whole series of reasons as outlined in Chapter 5. If you can come to understand your own vulnerability and the vital signs when you are likely to be susceptible, you can either avoid getting cold sores all together or reduce the frequency and scale of outbreaks.

4. Tingling

The first signs a cold sore is coming is with an itching or tingling sensation. It is normally accompanied by redness, slight swelling or heat. This will normally be when immunity is low. It can often be at bed time when you are less sharp and therefore miss this critical tell tale signs that one is coming. If you are tired, feeling unwell, under the weather, jetlagged, stressed, sun-struck or under the influence of alcohol the chances are you may not notice the tingling. Then you wake up with a cold sore. It can all happen very quickly. If you are lucky enough to catch the tingling phase (though you definitely won't feel lucky) you can head off the cold sore and stop it breaking out by following the steps in this book.

The tingling phase can be very hard to detect. After a number of outbreaks you start to think you have a cold sore coming when you don't. Once you truly understand your susceptibility then detecting the tingling phase becomes much more reliable. Then you kick yourself that you could have let you guard down by doing something that you should have known would risk triggering an outbreak.

5. Swelling

As mentioned, you will often notice the swelling when you wake up. Out of the blue you have a cold sore and it is no longer a tingle. It is ravaging, shinny, painful area of swollen redness and full of fluid and about to burst. Often there is a white spot (or series of spots) forming like a pimple where the blister will burst. Even at this late stage, I will show you how to stop the cold sore from bursting, blistering and scabbing. But we will look at how you can avoid even getting to this stage in the first place.

6. Blistering

So, then the bubble bursts with the fluid, which is highly contagious to others and other parts of your body. The best route to reducing a cold sore's worst effects is to avoid the blister bursting, but if it does we are then into a damage limitation exercise to reduce the size of the scab and speed up the healing which I will also cover.

7. Scabbing

This is the most visibly noticeable aspect of a cold sore. The dark penny piece on the lip that you can see in a mirror from a mile away. And therefore, you think others can too. The techniques outlined in this book will show you how to avoid getting a scab every time. I haven't had one myself in years now.

8. Healing

The scab can take seemingly ages to heal and drop off. Like any other scab on the body, it is around a week which seems an age when it is on your face. We will look at reducing healing time too, though this shouldn't be necessary as going forward you will be able to avoid getting a scab all together.

9. Scarring

Whatever you do, never squeeze a cold sore and always resist the temptation to pick a scab off. This will almost certainly leave some scarring. I unwittingly did both of these. I found ways to reduce the scarring. I will give you some tips on how to deal with this too.

10. Recovery

Once the cold sore has gone you skin in that area should make a full recovery. You may be left with a little redness for a while. It is important you don't aggravate the area by picking or scratching it. Remember that injury to the area can cause an outbreak as well. Your cold sore is gone for now, but you are back to step 2 in this life cycle.

It is said that around 80% of the population in the United States has HSV1. So, you are certainly not alone if you get cold sores. It's how you now deal with them that counts!

Genital Herpes (HSV2)

It is extremely important that you observe strict hygiene while you have a cold sore outbreak. HSV can be passed to your own genitals through contact. It can also be passed by contact with others, so during an outbreak abstain from touching your own genitals as best you can or other people's. This also applies if they have a cold sore outbreak. HSV-2 is most commonly spread via sexual contact, but there is a risk of spreading HSV to the genitals via oral sex.

So if either you, your partner or anyone else in your household has a cold sore. Wash hands thoroughly (I count to 15 while washing) and frequently, even before and after going to the bathroom and keep bath towels separate. A dedicated hand towel for your hand washing is also a good idea. Consider using a bacterial hand wash. See more on this under Hygiene in chapter 7.

This book is written for sufferers of HSV-1 and is based on my own experience. None of the treatments covered here are recommended for HSV-2. But, it is likely that the aspects of diet, learning about susceptibility to an outbreak and understanding the lysine-arginine balance will also be helpful to sufferers of HSV2.

4.   Products for treating cold sores

I reckon I have tried pretty much everything when it comes to treating cold sores. Here is a very brief summary of products I have used and my reaction to them. This is by no means a recommendation and equally where I have not had success, those products may work for you. We are all different.

Ice

One of the main reasons for updating this book to a second edition is that in recent years I have increasingly found that ice can dramatically reduce the scale of a cold sore. Sometimes it can stop a cold sore altogether. There are three methods I use, depending on what I have in the freezer. Each method requires you to hold the ice/frozen object in a towel to soak up the melted water. You also need to be careful that the ice/object will not stick to your skin on initial contact (avoid metals). Touch it on the back of your hand and let it melt a little first to reduce the risk of it sticking to your lips.

The sooner you can apply ice (i.e. at the very first signs/tingling) the better the outcome will be. There will be much less swelling, which in turn reduces the need for the cold sore to burst. With this technique, which we will discuss in more detail in Chapter 7, I have found I can go out and about within 24 hours.

The three forms of ice that I may use are:

- ice blocks from an ice tray
- frozen ice packs, normally used to keep a cool bag cold
- frozen containers – for me normally soup (see Diet in Chapter 5)

Creams

I have tried all of the products below. I have found most topical creams to have little effect at preventing a cold sore outbreak or reducing the cold sore once you have one. Most of these creams seem to be targeted at reducing the pain or cracking of the skin associated with a cold sore. One of the aspects of improved healing, covered in chapter 7, is keeping a wound moist. These creams may improve the healing process.

I generally use two. Zovirax is probably the market leader and has acyclovir (the anti-viral compound covered below) as its main active ingredient. It is a white cream which doesn't lend itself well to application once the skin is broken. It is also not good for disguising the sore unless you can rub it in with a little bit of finger pressure. This is why it lends itself well to the pre-blistering stage. I find it soaks into the skin well after the ice treatment mentioned above. Wash your hand thoroughly after application!

Lysine is covered in detail in the next chapter and I would favor the Lysine creams. My favorite one is Lip-Clear Lysine + by Quantum Health, available in most pharmacies in America and online in other countries. It is the best cold sore cream I have found by a long way. This is a herbal based cream and you only have to use a small amount. It is also a handy pocket-sized tube. I tend to use Zovirax if I think I have an outbreak coming as mentioned, in the hope that I might avoid it or lessen it. But I find Lip-Clear is better once I have avoided the breaking of a blister, as outlined in this book, I find that it reduces swelling and speeds up healing beneath the skin.

- **Lip-Clear Lysine +**
- **Zovirax**
- Blistex
- Cymex
- Super Lysine +
- Releev
- Abreva
- Anbesol
- Hubner Silicea Gel
- Campho-Phenique

If you can't find Lip-Clear Lysine + cream in your country, look online for another cream that contains Lysine.

Lip balms

There are a few lip balms available. Cold sores often come from over exposure to ultra-violet light in the sun's rays. So, protecting the area with a sun-screen with a good sun protection factor (SPF) is a good precaution. I sail and ski a lot and although I have had very few outbreaks that I would consider to be sun related, I always carry a tube of sun block when exposed to extreme sunlight. I simply apply it to area on my lip where I would normally get an outbreak. My favorite is Herpecin L and I normally have a few sticks of it hidden in various pockets of sailing and skiing jackets. If you cannot find this one, just use another SPF lip balm for protection.

People often share lip balms. I apply mine discretely away from other people to avoid being asked and then being faced with the awkwardness of explaining why it is best they don't. Equally, I decline using someone else's lip balm for fear of the risk of contaminating it.

I have probably only had a couple of cold sores in the early days from too much sun while sailing. I have not had any skiing, which might be down to the exercise. But I always remain cautious and I know several people for which sunburn is a dead cert for a cold sore outbreak.

Patches

Clear patches for covering a cold sore are becoming increasing available. I have tried Compeed cold sore patches several times. I know other sufferers who use a few patches to cover the whole cold sore area. The patches are not highly visible, though I think they are a bit shiny and the outline is detectable. They do protect the area. The real downside I found is that they can develop a wrinkle as the area may not be flat and then they can come off quite easily.

There are also new liquid patches emerging. One I have tried is Herpatch Cold Sore Serum. I was attracted to this because it appeared to be less rigid and a patch that would provide some degree of medication as well. My experience is that it wasn't as good as my preferred technique outlined in Chapter 7. Patches were instrumental in me finding my best way of dealing with cold sores and this did start me thinking about ways to medicate the covering of a cold sore as well.

Tablets

Lysine

Lysine tables are commonly available and using these is covered in detail in chapter 7. I have tried several brands from different pharmacies and health food shops. They mostly come as 500mg or 1000mg. The tablets don't taste that nice. Some come in capsule form which are a little easier to swallow. Either way, Lysine in tablet or capsule form all seem to be pretty much the same.

Antiviral

If you go to a doctor with your cold sore symptoms they will probably give you a prescription for Aciclovir (Acyclovir) which is an antiviral treatment. Doses vary from 200mg every few hours right up to 800mg with a course typically lasting two weeks. I tried these for a few years with increasing doses.

One of the problems I found was by the time I got to see the doctor to get a prescription the outbreak was well underway. The doctors were keen to point out that the tablets had a shelf life and were ineffective as a preventative measure. I also found I was suffering from mild side effects such as headaches. I became less and less comfortable using antiviral drugs personally, but in the end it is something you should discuss with your doctor.

In consulting my doctor at the time, I did get a growing sense that he felt that cold sores were just a fact of life and that once you have HSV, it is best to let cold sores take their own course. I guess that is an understandable reaction when seeing other patients with more serious medical illnesses, but I was determined to find my own way of dealing with cold sores and reducing the social impact for me personally.

Liquid Lysine

Quantum Health, the producers of my favorite lysine cream - Lip Clear Lysine +, also have a liquid lysine extract with Echinacea and shiitake mushroom extracts. It is a dietary supplement which can be added to water or tea. This is potentially a good alternative to tablets. The liquid also contains vitamin C, alcohol and distilled water. One other advantage of this liquid is that it dries quickly and can be applied to the cold sore in the tingling phase of a breakout before a blister forms. Because it dries in this way it can be applied before a patch and may reduce the scale of the outbreak.

Electronic Devices

The most common of these devices is a battery operated invisible light treatment device. I have tried a couple of these devices having seen people swear by them on the internet. I was up for trying anything, especially if it wasn't another form of medication. You cover the cold sore area with the device, press a button and for three minutes it emits a wavelength of light that is meant to dramatically reduce the healing time of a cold sore.

One common theme in many of the reviews is the device doesn't last very long, hence I tried two. But personally I have had not had much success with this product. Try it by all means and see if it helps. It maybe a useful added treatment to my preferred method outlined later. Anything that you can do early on to make the cold sore recede is worth trying and these products are meant to do that.

Heat treatment

Another device, Herpotherm, uses heat treatment and has fairly good reviews online. One of the problems that people also cite here is that the device doesn't last. I have also become more and more skeptical of internet reviews. Reading the responses to each review and the ensuing discussion can be insightful as well.

Other treatments

Toothpaste

I saw some reports that applying toothpaste on top of the cold sore can help. Two brands that contain stannous fluoride, discussed under Medavir below, are Crest and Oral B. If you are short of a lysine cream or can't get to a pharmacy, toothpaste may be better than nothing.

Red Marine Algae

It is said that red marine algae can assist the body's immune response to viruses. It is a sea vegetable that has many times the amount of minerals of land based plants. It is used to maintain a proper alkaline balance in the body, can be useful for weight loss and lowering cholesterol. In relation to HSV, it can reduce the number of outbreaks and their severity by reducing the formation of the virus colonies. I tried RMA tablets some years ago without much success, but as a supplement in times of vulnerability such as winter, they may prove useful as a regular supplement to reduce the likelihood of a cold sore outbreak.

Oxygen Therapy

There is a great deal on the internet about using oxygen or ozone to kill the bacteria that viruses thrive on. Most methods of increasing oxygen in the body are carried out by therapists. Food grade hydrogen peroxide is another treatment that is often cited as being able to kill the virus all together. It is pretty scary stuff as it burns your skin if you touch it. I tried this technique myself. I did the course of drops in water as recommended and it didn't work.

The 1931 Nobel prize winner, Dr. Otto Warburg, showed that cancer cells thrive in an oxygen deficient environment. With decades of research since this discovery, it is now well known that low blood oxygen levels are associated with people with chronic diseases. So the idea of treating the HSV virus this way may have some credibility. We will look at oxygenation of the blood further in the next chapter.

Medavir Stannous Fluoride Gel

I tried this product for a few years but it isn't readily available now. It claimed to reduce the quantity of the virus with regular treatment. I can't say this was true in my case but it was my first route to discovering the power of preventing the cold sore blister bursting. The stannous fluoride was meant to be the active ingredient and it may have reduced the scale of the swelling. There was certainly a burning sensation when applying it.

For me the really valuable aspect of the Medavir product was this sticky gel covering the spot and preventing an outbreak. The permanently sticky nature of the gel was not ideal as it was harder to disguise but it did lead me to thinking of using liquid bandage, which dries, as an alternative.

And lots of wives tales and miracles

If you look long and hard enough on the internet you will find scores of theories and remedies that are meant to work wonders. Some of these sound so plausible and compelling, but beware of any claims for completely curing the herpes simplex virus. If you do find a miracle cure yourself that does actually work, please let me know. But the general rule is that if it is too good to be true, it probably is.

5.   Know your vulnerability

The single best way to stop getting cold sores is to establish why you get
them in the first place. My experience is that different people get them
for different reasons. Once you truly understand your own vulnerabilities
and the conditions that normally trigger an outbreak, you are a long way
towards avoiding getting cold sores altogether.

Low immunity

Whatever the reason for an outbreak, the overwhelming evidence is that
the HSV virus attacks when your immune system is functioning lower than
normal. This can be for a host of reasons many of which are outlined
below. One of the real problems with this is actually knowing when your
immune system is low. There are not many obvious tell-tale signs.
Ironically one of the most cited tell-tale signs for low immunity is getting
cold sores. Others are getting colds, swollen glands, an infection or
recovering from a serious illness. The problem is low immunity almost
creeps up on you without you noticing and then it is too late.

Many of the triggers outlined in this chapter are the situations that lead to
low immunity in the first place. So, knowing what causes your own low
immunity is vital. Here are a few tips:

- Avoid infection by washing your hands regularly – count to 15
- Consider taking supplements such as Zinc or Airborne, especially
  in the winter months
- A deep tissue massage can increase immune boosting blood cells
  and reduce stress
- Probiotics such as yoghurt with friendly bacteria help boost the
  immune system
- Keep warm, it sounds obvious but try and avoid catching a chill or
  dramatic temperature change
- Make sure you get a good night's sleep - camomile tea can help
  you sleep
- Avoid too much fat, wheat and refined sugar in your diet - harder
  with a hangover
- Too much caffeine or alcohol will lower your immunity. Smoking is
  very bad for your immunity

- Exercise is also good for raising energy levels, expelling toxins and helping with sleep patterns
- Drink plenty of water to hydrate and flush toxins out of your system

Those are the things you should do, but here are just some of the signs that your immune system might be low:

- a slight sore throat or headache, the feeling you might be catching a cold
- needing a lot of coffee to stay awake or needing a drink to relax
- struggling to concentrate or to focus at work
- feeling irritable or annoyed with someone of something small

Exhaustion

A person's immunity can be at a low ebb due to exhaustion. This can be for one of the following reasons:

- Jet lag
- lack of sleep or burning the candle at both ends
- tiredness from speaking all day at a conference or exhibition
- heatstroke for too much sun exposure
- stress - problems at work or home

Some of these are more obvious than others. You may not notice you are physically or mentally exhausted and then it creeps up on you and can't stay awake or, worse still, collapse. Jet lag from long distance travel or heatstroke are a dangerous mix of tiredness and climatic change, which we will look at further in this chapter. Jet lag disrupts your body clock. You many not feel any effect on your immune system, but chances are you are at a much higher risk of getting a cold sore. I have often developed a cold sore after a long-haul flight. Weather this is down to temperature change or the jet lag, I don't know. What I do know is, that I need to boost my immune system. If you fly long haul to a conference in a much colder place, then you have a triple risk. See some of the perfect storm examples in the next chapter.

Diet

A poor diet is a big contributor to low immunity and heightened cold sore risk. Add junk food as an extra factor to flying long haul to a much colder place for a demanding conference or a grueling round of back to back meetings and you have a quadruple whammy. Add long nights out drinking and clubbing to top things off and you are almost guaranteed a cold sore in return. If you know this is what you are in for, then you can take some preventative action up front to prepare your immune system. Follow the tips outlined at the start of this chapter and look at some of the perfect storm examples in the next chapter.

It is definitely worth improving your diet in the run-up times of vulnerability once you know they are coming. In his excellent book, Super Immunity, Dr Joel Fuhrman explains how proper nutrition colds, flue and other infections. He goes right into the science and studies and covers anti-cancer super foods. Many of his tips on eating and sustaining a healthy diet also apply to suppressing viruses such as HSV.

Covering diet and nutrition in any detail is beyond the scope of this book but some key summary points I have learned from researching this area myself are below:

- green leaf vegetables - kale, watercress, spinach, Swiss chard are the highest nutrition foods
- cruciferous vegetables - broccoli, cauliflower, Brussels sprouts, bok choy are also very good
- carrots offer many benefits and are great for juicing
- berries - strawberries, blackberries, raspberries and blueberries are good nutritionally
- beans and lentils - these offer extra protein in a balance diet
- nuts and seeds - these are lower down the nutrition list - see the warning in the next section

There are increasing arguments against the nutritional value of animal-based foods such as meat, fish (farmed is especially bad), eggs (though, said to be one of the best food for immunity) and dairy (though high in lysine). Some studies are going further with outright health warnings, especially for red meat and processed meats. Whatever your view, there is little doubt that the highest nutritional foods are vegetables. For instance, Dr Fuhrman shows in his book, vegetables like kale, watercress and collards have a nutrition density index score of 1,000 verses around a value of only 30 for fish, eggs and dairy products. Most processed foods have an even lower score, so these deprive your immune system. Cruciferous vegetables, ones that have a four petal flower forming a cross, are shown to be especially beneficial for human health and wellbeing.

Eating as many of the foods listed above as you can as part of your normal daily diet will dramatically raise your overall immunity and this is essential in the lead up to times of vulnerability. Once you know your susceptibility to what triggers your cold sores, learn to up your nutrition intake with these foods.

Soups

Since writing the first edition of this book, I bought a soup-maker. I didn't even know such a thing existed until a friend told me about theirs. There is no easier and quicker way of getting a high nutrition diet. You simply add green leaf veg and chop up any root veg, throw in some stock, turn on the soup maker and come back 20 minutes later and you have delicious highly nutritious fresh soup. You will never buy a ready-made soup with all the accompanying additives again. Soup is very much a winter things for me, the time when I am most susceptible to getting a cold sore. If my immunity is low or set to be low or I sense a cold sore coming, I up my nutritional intake by making lots of soups with high nutrition foods.

One small tip, let your soup cool down so as to not risk burning your lips or the cold sore area and to make it easier to swallow each spoonful without the soup dribbling over your cold sore which will dirty the area or worse scold it.

The soup maker normally makes more soup than I can eat on one go, so I freeze what is left over. This means I have an immediate supply to boost my immunity when needed. But the best thing I have found by far is that I have plastic tubs of frozen soup which are ideal for my first line defense, ice treatment. See Chapter 7.

Lysine-Arginine balance

There is overwhelming evidence that cold sore outbreaks will occur if your balance of lysine to arginine, two amino acids, is too low. We will come to see that lysine supplements can be used to treat cold sores very effectively. But it is worth understanding which foods are high in lysine as well as the ones that are high in arginine. A comprehensive table of foods and their ratios is given in Appendix A, but it is worth noting the top foods that are high in each in this order.

Foods High in Lysine - Good	Foods High in Arginine - Bad
• Margarine	• Nuts - walnuts, pine nuts and hazelnuts
• Yoghurt	• Orange juice
• Cheese	• Grapes
• Papaya (paw paw)	• Berries
• Beets (beetroot)	• Onions, Garlic
• Butter, Milk, Cream, Ice cream	• Rice, Seeds
• Mango, Apricot, Apple	• Cereals - Oats, Corn, Wheat, Bran

Are you nuts?!

Nuts are the worst food you can eat to bring on cold sores. Walnuts, hazelnuts and pine nuts are through the roof with more than 5 times as much arginine than lysine. Orange juice is the next worst thing, also a ratio greater than 5. There is a long list of other nuts and some seeds like sesame around 4 to 1, followed by grapes and blackberries and blueberries at 3 to 1. Then foods such as onions, garlic and cereals come in over 2 to 1.

In his brilliant book, The Four Hour Body, Tim Ferris describes nuts as 'domino foods.' Foods that are not too detrimental to a diet in small quantities, but it can be hard to stick to eating small quantities because they can be so addictive. Once you start it is hard to stop. If you have HSV1, then you have to accept nuts are a high-risk food. If you must eat them, very small quantities and definitely not during times of vulnerability.

I love nuts, but I have increasingly come to the conclusion I need to avoid them all together in the winter. If I am in a bar and the bartender puts them in front of me, I tell them I am allergic (which is kind of true) and ask them to take them away.

Get into dairy and a few fruits

Margarine is the highest lysine food with a ratio to arginine of 3 to 1. But realistically eating tubs of margarine is not an exciting prospect. The good news is that yoghurt comes a very close second and that is easy to eat lots of once you get into it. Nearly all cheeses are good, especially Swiss cheese, at close to 3 to 1. Beets (beetroot) are 2.5 to 1 and most other dairy is over 2 to 1. Mango, apricots and apples also come in at 2 to 1. One tip on eating apples. It can be a strain on the cold sore area opening your mouth wide to take the first bite of the apple and there is a risk of juice running over the sore. Cut your apple up into pieces first to make eating the apple easier. For the prefect combo add pieces of apple, mango or apricot to your yogurt.

Concentrations are important

It is not just the ratio that counts. The quantities present in normal sized portions of food is also important. For example 100g of walnuts has 2.5g of arginine, while 227g of plain yoghurt has only 0.7g of lysine. If you ate these two portions you would consume less than 1.2g or lysine and 2.7g of arginine. Put it another way, you need to eat half a kilo (1 lb) of yoghurt to only 100g of walnuts, 5 times as much, just to balance your lysine/arginine intake. Of course to avoid getting cold sores, an even balance is not really enough. We need to tip the scales well in favor of lysine.

In Appendix A, I have also added a table for the amount of lysine per 100g portion ranked highest to lowest. If you think of 100g as typically a handful, then it is easier to appreciate the amount of lysine and arginine you are consuming in terms of milligrams per handful. The ratios are still important, but this gives you an understanding of how much of a food you need to consume to get a like for like intake of lysine.

So, we see cheese and milk score highly with very favorable ratios. This means you have to eat a lot more yoghurt to get the same amount of lysine as you would eating cheese. Remember, that with the metric scale, 100g (3.5 oz or half a cup of sugar) of water equals 100ml (3.5 fl oz or just under half a cup of water). So, with a liquid like milk that's a quarter of a soda can's worth. At the bottom of this table, while we see apples have a good ratio over 2 to 1, you only get 10mg of lysine per 100g versus around 3000mg per 100g for cheese. You would need to eat enough apples to make yourself sick to get close to matching a handful of cheese in terms of lysine intake.

So, a really simple tip, ahead of or, during a cold sore outbreak is - Eat lots of Swiss Cheese!

Avoiding arginine when you are vulnerable

There is a table in Appendix A for the amount of arginine. Here we see pine nuts (also a main ingredient in pesto) come top at almost 5g per 100g, a very high concentration and almost twice that of walnuts. Peanuts and peanut butter (which is recommended in a lot of diets and something I love to eat straight off the spoon) are lethal when it comes to arginine as are seeds.

The food equivalent to lysine tablets

It is also worth noting the amount of food that equates to a 500mg lysine tablet, the off the shelf standard. So, there is a forth table in the appendix which shows the weight of food portion you need to eat to achieve the same lysine intake. There will be some arginine present in lysine heavy foods, but foods with good ratios contain 500mg of lysine for the following amounts:

Cheese 15g to 30g (30g = 1oz)
Fish 20g to 30g
Meat 30 to 50g

Most vegetables, which are essential for proper immune function, hover around a ratio of one to one - lysine to arginine neutral. These tables in Appendix A are a useful searchable reference.

So, the simple advice is: at times of vulnerability, **don't eat nuts**, berries or seeds and **eat lots of dairy**, especially cheese and yoghurt.

Oxygenation and Exercise

We mentioned oxygen therapy in the last chapter as being a significant factor for suppressing viruses. Our health depends largely on how efficiently nutrients can be absorbed and utilized at a cellular level and how well toxins can be removed. Waste and toxins are removed through the normally bodily functions of filtration via the kidneys and liver and excreted in urine or bowels as well as by perspiration. The more toxic poisons in the body are eliminated via oxidation a process of oxygen rich red blood cells circulating in the body. Ways to ensure the right oxygen balance in your body include:

- alkaline diet - more plant based, less processed and animal based foods
- adequate hydration - drinking enough water - especially filtered and ionized water
- breathing exercises - have been cited as being helpful, meditation and yoga can help
- daily exercise - especially aerobic exercise such as walking or cycling

After getting the right amount sleep and eating a healthy diet, exercise is the most important factor for a healthy immune system. Just a good brisk walk or bike ride for twenty minutes every day will be beneficial to your overall health. Doing this in fresh clean outdoor air may also prove more beneficial than a workout in a gym full of air that is re-circulated via air conditioning.

Testing your oxygen level

There is a basic test which is popular among doctors in Russia known as a Control Pause or CP test. This involves relaxing for five minutes or so and then pinching your nose and holding after a normal breath out with your mouth closed. While doing this you measure the seconds before you experience the first desire to breath. This is not a measure of how long you can hold your breath, but more when you become uncomfortable -

i.e. an involuntary push of the diaphragm or a swallowing in your throat. When you release you should be able to resume your normal breathing pattern before you pinched your nose.

Doctor Buteyko, who developed the test found that the results on over 250,000 people generally held that:

- 1-10 seconds = severely sick, critically or terminally ill
- 10-20 seconds = sick patients with health complaints, often on daily medication
- 20-30 seconds = people with average health, no serious health problems
- 40-60 seconds = very good health
- over 60 seconds = ideal health, chronic disease virtually impossible

I became interested in this test myself because I found it so hard to know or find some kind of measure for when my immune system function was low. This doesn't measure your immunity as such, but given nutrition, hydration, breathing and exercise all contribute to your oxygen levels, this might be a useful way of knowing if you are above or below par. I think knowing your normal level is key and then understanding any fluctuations from it. I simply remember the 20 second boundary. Below it, I am not in full health, above it I am average. Plus or minus 10 seconds are my outer bands for good and bad. I have found that for the rare times I get a cold sore coming, I am below 20 seconds with this test. Now when I am worried about my vulnerability, I run the test. It is enough to prompt me to go for a walk getting lots of fresh air, eat well, take some lysine and get a good night's sleep with the window open if possible.

Climate

Cold sores are so named as they are associated with catching a cold. They are sometimes called fever blisters as in catching a fever. Given catching a cold or fever is associated with a low immune system this is a reasonable assumption, but evidence suggests cold sores can be associated with a series of climatic changes or events.

Big changes in temperature

I have found that if I travel somewhere that is over 15 degrees C (60F) colder I am highly susceptible to getting a cold sore. I ski a great deal and strangely I have not had a cold sore on a ski trip (touch wood). I put this down to one of two things. Either its is because I am getting exercise which helps the immune system and oxygenation. Or it is because I am always fearful and take preventative measures. I do know of people who consistently get cold sores when they go skiing, so the risk is there. Again it about knowing there is a risk and where your own susceptibility is greatest.

Many people report getting a cold sore in the winter when temperatures start to fall. I find I am particularly vulnerable in the fall or during a cold spell in the spring. Looking at ways to boost your immune system around these times is important. if you feel you are getting a cold you are also probably at risk of getting a cold sore. I have often had a breakout just from catching a chill.

Air conditioning

I spent a long time thinking I only got cold sores in the winter. One summer in New York City, it was so hot for a few days that I went to bed with the air con on full blast. I woke up in the morning in a freezing room and bingo, I had a cold sore. I am now always careful not to catch a chill in air-conditioned offices and carry a sweater just in case. This only ever happened once, but once is enough to prove susceptibility. Extremes in temperature again was a cause in this instance.

Sun – ultra-violet light

A lot of people get cold sores from too much sun exposure. UV light brings them out. I sail a lot so this susceptibility would be a nightmare for me. After years of thinking I didn't get cold sores from the sun, I finally got one after way too much unprotected exposure which is magnified by reflection at sea. It was a yacht race of several hours where I couldn't escape the sun. I haven't had one since and I mostly put that down to being very careful to cover the area with a lysine UV SPF lip balm. Given that snow reflects UV light, I now also use the same lip balm when I am skiing.

Vitamin D, associated with sunlight, is good for immune support so the right amount of sun exposure can be beneficial when absorbed by the body overall. Still cover the area where you get a cold sore to protect the area from UV exposure. Sunstroke also has an effect on your immune system. Wearing a hat (Tilley Hats are great as they shade your mouth area) and sun cream will help.

Given how many people report getting a cold sore outbreak when they get sunburnt, this is a definite risk you need to be aware of. Sweating is a sign as well and the pores will open more. Use an SPF lip balm.

Humidity

I hadn't heard of this one until it was too late. I had an outbreak once after travelling to Chicago from Europe so the cold and jet lag may have been contributing factors. I remembered feeling tired from talking to people at a conference all day and felt I would grab a quick sauna at the hotel in order to warm up and de-stress. Later that night at dinner, I felt the cold sore coming on. Because I constantly want to know why I got one to establish my own susceptibility, I asked myself 'what have I done in the past 24 hrs?' and then searched 'cold sores sauna' on the internet and sure enough people had reported getting them.

It seams that the humid conditions that accompany saunas, steam rooms, hot tubs and long hot baths or showers may open the pores to create a gateway for the virus to want to escape. That night I would have been best to fit a short sleep in when I was feeling tired. Now, if I am run down, I am conscious that taking a sauna is a risk. Saunas may also be detrimental to oxygenation, although ironically special ozone saunas are one form of oxygen therapy.

Another observation is I once caught a cold sore in Singapore which is a very humid place. I had been walking outside but it was cloudy, so I was surprised to later develop a cold sore. There is always more UV in the tropics than you think, even on cloudy days. But after the sauna experience a long time later, I put developing the cold sore that time in Singapore down to combination of humidity and UV exposure. I also slept in a heavily air-conditioned room that evening. Once you know your susceptibility, you avoid exposing yourself to that same set of conditions. I should have worn a hat and some UV lip balm and put the fan on instead of the air con.

Lip balm as a risk

While lip balms can protect you from UV exposure to the area, people have reported that their lip balms seem to make them vulnerable to getting a cold sore. So, you may need to look at changing should this happen. In very hot countries Zinc can provide a full block and visibly having your lips covered is acceptable.

The lip balm I like the most is Herpicin HL 30. It is SPF 30 and I put a big splodge on my lower lip where I get cold sores. People often point out I have slipped with my lip balm or sun block. I brush it off by saying I burn on my lower lip or maybe just make it a bit less obvious. I haven't had a cold sore if I have used this. It is recommended for use once you have a cold sore, or one coming. I think it is an effective preventer and it has worked for me so far and I always carry it in my pocket in the summer.

Surgery or Trauma to the area

This is another documented reason for getting a cold sore. Given the opening of pores already described under humid conditions can create a vulnerability, it is conceivable that any stress to the area might also do this. A fat lip from an impact, a cut from shaving. Be careful with blades razors during and soon after a cold sore outbreak and at times of vulnerability. Have a wet shave with a blade by all means, but consider using an electric razor over the usual outbreak area.

A bump, dental work or surgery may also increase vulnerability. If you have bitten your lip by accident, it may be enough to bring out a cold sore so prepare to take defensive action.

Kissing

Many people site a long night of kissing as being the precursor to an outbreak. Of course kissing is by far the most likely route for contracting the HSV1 virus in the first place and if you get cold sores you will be wary of long nights kissing for fear of the risk of an outbreak and passing on to someone. Prolonged kissing could be considered as a form of trauma to the area, but it is probably unlikely that kissing on its own brings on cold sores. If you are already vulnerable with low immunity, poor diet, temperature change, sun exposure or humidity - chances are that kissing is the final icing on the cake that triggers a cold sore forming. Tiredness from a long night out drinking and clubbing, sitting outside or getting cold stripping off, followed by hours of passion are the more likely set of conditions leading to a cold sore here.

Hormonal changes

Many women report that they get cold sores with hormonal changes when premenstrual or pregnant. These vulnerabilities are clearly not easily avoided, but they are for the most part predictable.

What we are coming to see is that cold sores often come with a combination of factors and improving immune function, diet and avoiding contributing climatic factors will reduce vulnerability at these times.

6.   The perfect storm - Avoiding an outbreak

Learning the conditions that make you vulnerable to a cold sore attack is vital to reducing the number and severity of outbreaks in the future. It may take many outbreaks before you work out your own vulnerability. It took me years. Hopefully this book will dramatically reduce the time it takes you to work it out for yourself.

When you get an outbreak, record the likely causes covered in the last chapter and why they existed. Start to look at an outbreak as the opportunity to avoid getting a cold sore next time. It is quite likely that there was a combination of factors that created the perfect storm for an outbreak.

Here are a few scenarios and some tips on how to avoid allowing the perfect storm conditions to allow a cold sore to develop.

You are feeling exhausted

Look at cancelling plans to go out. Stay inside and avoid the cold. Take a break from drinking alcohol and get a couple of early nights where you can sleep around 10 hours. Substitute drinking caffeine for herbal tea. Avoid nuts and eat some cheese if you can. Take a couple of lysine tablets as a precaution. Avoid hot baths, saunas and air conditioning. If your immune system is already low, exercise may now be detrimental. Rest is key.

You are flying long haul

Get your diet in order in the run up to the flight and catch up on sleep before you travel as well. Try and avoid the red eye flight or one that arrives very late at night. Avoid nuts and drinking alcohol on the flight and reduce caffeine intake. Avoid dehydration from flying, drink lots of water. Treat yourself to a cab to where you are staying. Always keep the first night of your arrival for yourself. If I am visiting old friends, especially if it is cold, I often check in to a hotel for my first night. Go to bed early. Resist the hotel sauna, gym and spa and consider a long walk in the fresh air instead. Try and eat healthily during your travels. I often do a shop at Whole Foods just to keep a better handle on my diet. Take lysine in the run up to and during your trip.

You are under a lot of stress

You may have an exam coming or be under pressure at work. You may not feel stressed, but look out for the signs - irritability, biting finger nails, chewing pencils, unable to sleep etc. Keeping your immunity up by eating well is essential. Again, avoid the cold, nuts and drinking alcohol. If you are needing caffeine to stay awake this is a sure sign you are in need of rest as well. Take lysine and walks in the fresh air.

The weather is turning cold

If the leaves are changing color and you are feeling a sore throat or cold coming on. You are quite literally, under the weather. Get lots of sleep. Eat well. Avoid nuts and take lysine tablets for a while.

You are speaking at a conference

You might be doing a presentation, which has been a bit of a stress in the run up to it. You may have spent the whole day on your feet speaking to people at an exhibition in an airless venue. You have been drinking coffee all day and not had a moment to stop. Perhaps you missed lunch and are exhausted. Avoid nuts. Avoid going out, especially if it is cold. Skip the night out partying with clients and get a good night's sleep. Take some lysine tablets.

You have got too much sun

You are clearly sunburnt or feeling very tired from a long day in the sun. you may not know it, but you have sunstroke which has run your immune system down. Avoid the temptation to cool down for the night with the air con on full blast. Stay off nuts, alcohol and caffeine. Eat well and get a good night's sleep. Take some lysine tablets.

You have an injury or infection

This could be a trauma to your mouth after the dentist, a fat lip, a bitten
lip or another wound somewhere else on your body. You may just be
fighting a cold. You may be fighting an illness such as bad back or sore leg.
Maybe your liver is not functioning properly, or you are just feeling out of
sorts. Either way, you are probably vulnerable. Eat well, rest well and take
some lysine tablets as a precaution.

You are experiencing hormonal changes

If you are a woman you may have your period coming. Another sure sign
is that your skin is breaking out in more spots or acne than usual. Again,
you are vulnerable and all the same rules of avoiding adding another
compounding factor apply and protecting yourself.

Be Prepared

The first signs of a cold sore coming normally catches sufferers completely
off guard. They are shocked and had no idea they were vulnerable. Even if
you are able to spot one of the above 'perfect storm' conditions you can
be caught out. Once you know you have a cold sore coming your stress
levels will inevitably increase. It can be self for-filling. Working out what
caused it and removing some uncertainly can help.

At the end of the next chapter I explain how to prepare your own cold
sore treatment kit. There is nothing worse than being caught out without
the ability to act in the face of a cold sore coming. Being able to deal with
it will reduce your stress levels which in itself will help reduce the scale of
the outbreak. Most of all you should be able to contain it avoid a blister
forming with the right kit and that in itself will make you feel a lot better.

Avoiding getting cold sores in the first place is the aim, but if all else fails
dealing with an outbreak to minimize the effects is your next line of
action.

7.   Dealing with an outbreak

Once you get to know your vulnerability, you start to build a sense of what you need to do ahead of the time you are most likely to get an outbreak. It may take several outbreaks for you to truly understand your vulnerability and even once you do there may be the rare occasion where you are caught off guard and the virus attacks.

Tingling

The first signs of an outbreak come from feeling a tingling or itching in the area you normally get a cold sore. For the vast majority of sufferers this is on or around the lip. It seems that all references talk about this tingling feeling as something where it is easy to spot the signs, but in reality it can be hard to sense clearly. You end up developing a paranoia that you have a cold sore coming. You check in the mirror and can't see anything. It is often a false alarm. Coupled with this, cold sores typically come at times when your awareness isn't great. You might be exhausted and not so alert to an outbreak. You may have had too much sun and feeling a bit weary as a result. Cold sores often start in the middle of the night and you wake up to find you have one coming, or worse it has arrived. Big Time!

Alcohol deserves special mention here and I guess this applies to drug use as well. Chances are, you contracted the HSV1 virus while kissing someone while under the influence of alcohol. There still isn't enough education on how to avoid getting the virus. I wish I had known more about it before I contracted it. There aren't many references on how to avoid catching cold sores.

I strongly recommend abstaining from drinking alcohol during periods of your vulnerability or an outbreak. If you are vulnerable with low immune system function, alcohol definitely won't help. You will be less aware of your vulnerability and do silly things like eating a bowl of nuts put in front of you at the bar. Most of all you will almost certainly miss the tingling sensation that precedes a cold sore outbreak if you have been drinking or are suffering a hangover. Drinking will delay any healing process. Worse still, you will be less aware of passing the virus to others or other parts of your body.

Visual signs with tingling

Once you know your vulnerability, you will check more regularly for visual signs of a cold sore coming in the mirror. Quite often it will be just your paranoia, but then one time you will spot it. You have a cold sore coming. If it is very early the surface will not have broken, but you can see a white or clear fluid building under the skin. Otherwise it may be redness or a slight swelling. If it is in the place you normally get cold sores, then chances are you have one coming. If the skin is unbroken you can press your finger lightly on this area and you may feel its a bit harder, like a lump in your lip. Whatever you do, do not squeeze this area at all. I did this the first time and I am sure my cold sores became worse as a result. If you are lucky enough to catch the cold sore at this very early stage, where there is no change to the surface of the skin, then you can almost certainly prevent an outbreak.

Apply ice as soon as possible!

I have found the basic rule of thumb is that the sooner you can get ice onto the sore area and the longer you can do it for, the more chance you have of avoiding an outbreak. If you are travelling, get some ice in a bucket in your hotel room. Failing that, get to a supermarket and buy the densest frozen food (like a liquid) you can find.

In my freezer at home, I always have:

- ice blocks, in bags or in an ice tray
- frozen ice packs, normally used to keep a cool bag cold
- frozen containers – for me normally soup

With any of these, remove the frost layer first in your hand or allowing a little initial melting. This will stop the frozen surface sticking to your skin. With a towel hold the ice/frozen object on the cold sore area. Ice melts quickly. Freezer packs are better, but a frozen tub container full of soup is ideal. A frozen plastic bottle of water would also work almost as well.

I find I can hold it in a towel to reduce the thaw, sit up or lie on my bed with it resting/balancing on my lip while reading. Rotating the tub so that a new colder frozen area is making contact seems to have the maximum effect.

How long should you do it for? This will depend on the severity or degree to which the sore has started. Because I nearly always want to avoid an outbreak at any cost and it always seems to be at the most inconvenient time, I will apply the freeze for as long as possible. Typically I will lie for an hour with the tub while reading or looking at my screen, watching TV etc. Then I will go and look in the mirror to see if it has gone down. The freezing will make the area look redder but hopefully it will be less swollen. It is as if the freezing is sending a signal to the virus to go away. I find this is also a good time to rub in some Zovirax cream (see below).

If after an hour, the swelling comes back I will give another freeze a go. I often have a couple of frozen soup tubs in the freezer so I can alternate. I may do this before bed and when I wake early in the morning, I may need to give it another go. If I catch the 'tingle' really early, one freeze might be enough. If not, it may take several goes. But either way, this will almost certainly stop the cold sore from breaking out, swelling and bursting.

With my most recent one, I felt a tingling during a night out drinking (one of many parties) just before Christmas. I went to the washroom, looked in the mirror and sure enough I could see a very small bubble developing. I probably would have spotted it hours earlier if I was at home, which would have been better. So, with no time to waste, I said my goodbyes and went home and did two tubs of ice which numbed the area. I was shattered, a sure sign of being run down, and went to bed and fell asleep. When I woke the next morning the swelling had come back a little but not as bad so I did a couple more freezes.

The pre-swelling of the cold sore tends to pucker or loosen the skin such that it is thinner and more fragile. So, you may reach a point where applying the ice will no longer be viable. If you have caught the swelling early enough, the sore will not develop and blister. You may just have to disguise a bit of redness. But if the skin is very lose, you will probably need to progress to applying the liquid skin as set out below.

In this recent instance, I applied some creams next day and managed to hide the unbroken sore (see below) and went out with friends. In the past, my lip would have blown up like a balloon at this stage. The following day, Christmas Day, I managed to disguise the last bit of redness again and no one even noticed anything in bright daylight. The next day, I applied some lysine cream just to aid full healing and the cold sore was as good as gone/never happened. This compares to what would have been two weeks in the past with me being a hermit for two weeks and cancelling New Years Eve parties.

Throughout this, I also took lysine tablets with a big dose when I got home having discovered the breakout. I should have been taking them already really and may have avoided a breakout all together.

What you need from the pharmacy

Here is a short list of things that you need from the pharmacy in order of importance:

1.   Liquid bandage - normally next to plasters
2.   Lysine tablets - 500mg or 1000mg - normally in the supplements section or in a health foods shop
3.   Q tips or cotton buds - often near cosmetics
4.   A Lysine cream - normally in the cold sore treatment section
5.   A makeup stick – can be very handy for disguising skin redness

You can survive with just the first one. If you cannot find this then cold sore patches are the next best thing, followed by the cold sore cream. If you can't find these then antiseptic cream will have to suffice. The first two items are the most important, the last three are nice to haves.

Next line of treatment

So, you have a cold sore coming as a result of one or more of the conditions we have outlined and you have applied the ice. Normally the symptoms you have reached are irreversible now. They've happened. The ice is your best chance at holding things at bay. The other thing that you can change quite quickly is your Lysine-Arginine balance. If you were aware of your vulnerability, you will probably have been taking Lysine tablets. But now you have a cold sore coming, this clearly hasn't been enough and you will need to consider upping your dose for a short time. How much is the right amount? I was at a point where I would consider swallowing the whole bottle of tablets if it would stop me getting a cold sore. Don't do this! You need to establish your minimum effective dose. That is the point where taking any more will have no additional benefit and could be detrimental to your health.

After some experimentation, I have found that a single large dose of around 3,000mg (6 x 500mg) is about the right amount for me. I stress, the right dose for me. I take 4 to 6 500mg tablets when I first notice I have a cold sore coming. This normally has a dramatic effect considerably reducing the size of the cold sore the next day. Dose is usually based on body weight. If you are younger, a woman, petite or taking Lysine for the first time try a smaller dose until you can establish the right amount for you. After your initial does you can then decrease back to 1,000mg a day over a couple of says and then 500mg or nothing a few days after that. If you are unsure or have other pre-existing medical conditions, please make sure you consult your doctor.

How safe is Lysine?

Some studies suggest that Lysine is more effective at preventing an outbreak than reducing the severity and duration of a cold sore outbreak. Keeping your lysine levels higher with a high lysine/low arginine diet while you are vulnerable is probably the best strategy. Lysine tablets can help in this vulnerability phase too. I have found that the increased dose with the very early signs can have a big impact.

For adults over 13 years the daily recommended dose is 12mg per kilogram of body weight per day (5 mg/lb). So, for an adult male weighing 85kg (187lb) that is 1000mg. During a flare up recommended doses range from 3,000 to 9,000mg per day taken in divided doses for a short period of time. I would never take 9,000mg and am happy with the lower end of that range.

Precautions

If you are on other medications, you need to consult your doctor. There is always potential for side effects and interactions with these and you should take dietary supplements such as Lysine under the supervision of a knowledgeable health care professional. Lysine in the diet is considered safe but high doses have been known to cause gallstones. There have also been reports of renal dysfunction, including Fanconi's syndrome and renal failure. People with kidney or liver disease should always ask their doctor before taking supplemental lysine. Pregnant and breastfeeding women should not take supplemental lysine without talking to their doctor.

Anecdotally, I know people who have taken lysine tablets and come out in lots of spots. If I have taken a high dose of lysine and avoided an outbreak. I drink lots of water with freshly squeezed lemon or lime to flush out my liver. If your liver function is below par lysine may also be less effective. This is another reason for cutting down your alcohol intake.

Lysine Creams

As well as taking Lysine tablets, you can also surround the area with a Lysine cream. I outline the ones I have tried in chapter 4. I have had the best results with Lip Clear Lysine by Quantum Health which is readily available in US pharmacies.

If the cold sore is coming and I am confident it won't burst overnight, I rub a little cream (normally Zovirax at this stage) lightly over the spot where the cold sore will come. I then add a good dab on top of this to be drawn into the skin for good measure. This is not very attractive so it is only really possible before bed or if you have elected to stay at home for the day. This first day is crucial.

The Sore Developing

With the ice treatment, the lysine tablets and cream applied at an early stage, you should manage to avoid an outbreak all together and the swelling will go down and within a day or two you will be back to normal, rather than the several days or couple of weeks it normally takes. But the treatment may not be enough and you could still get a small outbreak. You may not have caught the tingling early enough and you can now see that you are going to get a breaking of the skin and a blister. In my case I get a small white spot, pimple or indent emerging and this is where we need to deploy our next line of treatment.

To scab or not to scab?

There are differing views on this. Some healthcare professionals will advocate to just let the outbreak happen, let the scab develop and heal naturally in its own time. But the scab is the most visible aspect of a cold sore. It is normally dark red in color, raised and hard to disguise. It gets very itchy and the risk of scratching it, knocking it off and scaring is there as well. We will look at how best to treat a scar if this happens.

There is another very good reason for not allowing a blister to form and a scab to develop and that is the risk of spreading the virus to others or other parts of your body.

Preventing the blister from bursting

Sometimes it is hard to know if the ice and Lysine treatment has done enough to prevent a blister developing. This is something that you get better at judging. The developing spot is my tell-tale sign and I normally wait for that before resorting to this next step, but there are times where I don't bother with the Lysine cream and go straight to this next phase. This is typically for the following reasons:

1. It is bed time and I am not sure how things will develop in the night. A good night's sleep is also essential. It is worth cancelling engagements the following morning if you can and forewarning work you may be late in. Not having to stress about an early start will help. Also protecting the area from scraping it in bed is also a good idea.
2. I have to go to work or a meeting which I can't easily get out of. So a blob of cream sitting on my lip is not an option.

The one downside of preventing the blister from bursting is that you may get more swelling and a bit more pain in the early stages as the fluid is unable to escape. But the ice treatment should have reduced this considerably. If not, this swelling only lasts about a day versus the week of a scab healing.

Shaving and Showering

Men who have a cold sore coming, can not safely use a blade razor. Even if you're not a fan of electric razors you will need to get one. Bristles will be an obstruction for this next phase. With the electric razor, glide very gently over the cold sore area applying no pressure. Even these protected blades can eat into the sore if you are not careful. It can be better to shave before showering rather than after when the skin becomes too soft. When showering, be careful not to let the water jets hit the cold sore area directly. This especially applies with a scab as well for the risk of prematurely removing it and scaring. Generally, I try not to wash the area in the shower as tempting as it is to let water run over it. When drying after the shower you need to take extra care. I find it is best not to use the towel on the lower half of my face. I don't want to open the skin while it is soft and then risk spreading it. Also just in case it has opened up in the shower fluid might have run down the chin.

So, with a wet mouth area and chin, it is best to finish drying of with a tissue around the sore area. Then with a fresh tissue, just hold it lightly with one hand either side and lower onto the sore. If you have used lysine cream, this is the best way to remove the residue of cream to dry out the area. If the area is still not fully clean a very light dab with an alcohol swab is one way of ensuring it is. If you don't have a swab, a q-tip (cotton bud) run under the hot tap and rolled gently over the sore area to lift any residue is another possibility. After drying carefully with tissue or q-tip. It is best to let this area fully dry uncovered for a few more minutes.

When you return to the mirror with the area clean and dry, you will know for sure if you your cold sore has made it through the surface of the skin. If the Lysine treatment has been effective and you did get some fluid build up under the skin which is now receding, your skin will be stretched. If you place your tongue behind your lip and push it out very gently and back again you will notice how the skin tightens and then loosens.

Cold sore patches

In recent years several brands of small almost invisible patches to go over the sore have come onto the market. If you haven't got any fluid coming out of the sore these will work quite well. If the area is not fully dry, these will have trouble sticking. For me the patches are not ideal. I am conscious when I have one on that they are visible. They can come off. If you have the tell-tale spot developing, they won't stay on due to the irregular surface. In this instance they sort of pucker and wrinkle with an air bubble. They don't disguise very well with make up, though the manufacturers say they do. But perhaps their biggest drawback is they are a fixed size. I have seen some people using three in a row for example. But normally they are actually too big when compared with the technique I have discovered below.

If your cold sore has blistered or burst

The technique below is best to prevent a blister bursting and therefore scabbing, but it can be used if you are in the early stages of a burst blister. This means that you have only just noticed it has burst.

The first sign that a cold sore has blistered and burst is a very small droplet or series of droplets that look like sweat on the skin surface. You will probably first notice this after showering as described above. If this has happened, hold a clean piece of tissue across the area and look for fluid coming through the tissue in the mirror, or on the tissue when you pull it away. Hopefully you have caught the sore before this has happened and there is no fluid coming out.

Liquid Bandage - the miracle cure for cold sores

Another great innovation in recent years is liquid bandages. The idea of using these to prevent a cold sore outbreak came to me from using the Medavir Stannous Fluoride gel that I outlined in chapter 4 and the patches. The problem with the gel was that it was too sticky and runny. It needed a lot of re-applying and it was difficult to disguise with something like make up. While it was great that you could prevent an outbreak and scab, you just had this wet shinny lip for a few days where you could see the swelling underneath. At the other extreme the patches were too dry and didn't bond so well to the skin.

When I first saw liquid bandages in the pharmacy, I thought they would work. They are designed to cover and protect wounds. They go wet then dry and bond really well to the skin. It's flexible and waterproof and allows the skin to breath. There are lots of different brands that all seem to be much the same: New Skin, Skin Shield, Top Care, Nexcare, Germaline and pharmacy own brands. On the pack they say they prevent blisters and calluses, exactly what I was trying to achieve. The liquid also contains antiseptic which also aids healing and helps to prevent infection. But the biggest advantages of liquid bandages when it comes to cold sores is that you can apply exactly the right amount and they are really easy to disguise from even the closest viewer.

Applying liquid bandage to the area

Before you apply liquid bandage to the cold sore area it is worth experimenting somewhere else first. If you have a spot or mole on your hand or arm, try covering it really accurately. You will probably discover that you don't need as much as you would think to coat such a small area.

When it comes to covering a cold sore there are two key things. The first is, that unlike testing on your hand, you are now having to deal with gravity down the vertical surface of your face. Even just one drop of liquid bandage on the brush will turn out to be too much as it runs below the sore. And once it dries it is quite hard to get off. Don't worry we will look at how best to do this shortly, but it is best to get the coverage right first time. The second thing is you don't have to cover the whole cold sore area, just the point where it will (or has) burst. In fact it is best not to cover the whole area because you will come to see the edges of the liquid skin can pull away from the skin especially if you are using Lysine cream as well, which you can around the spot that you have put a very small amount of liquid bandage.

The other thing with liquid bandage is you can build up layers, so it is best to start very small and build from there. I find the brush that comes with it is ideal for applying it. But, just like a paint brush, if you have too much paint on, it will run everywhere. If you see a drip running down the stalk of the brush, you need to scrap it on the lip of the bottle so that it doesn't end up on your face. Lightly run the brush across the spot and wait for the first application to dry before you see if you need to build up more of a layer.

A word of caution, the liquid bandage might sting a little initially and also the instructions recommend you don't inhale it or swallow it. You need to be careful. Again, if you are unsure about this, consult your doctor.

This use of liquid bandage assumes your blister is not producing fluid from beneath the skin. If you are seeing fluid, remember that it is very contagious to others and other parts of your body. Also, you do not want to contaminate the liquid bandage fluid when you put the brush back in the bottle. In this instance it is best to use a new Q-tip with each application and dispose of it right away. If a lot of fluid is being produced from the sore, use one Q-tip to dry it and the other to apply the liquid bandage before more fluid comes out.

Once you have it covered, check after a while to see that it has held. With a burst blister, stopping it weeping is your first priority. Once this is done, go to the start of this chapter and follow the Lysine treatment with tablets.

Disguising the liquid bandage

The good news is that covering the point where the blister has or might burst should only be about a pin-prick in size. So that makes it easier to disguise and you may decide not to at all. Quite often the swelling is accompanied by redness around the area you have covered, and disguising it, is as much about covering this as it is hiding the liquid bandage.

I have found the best way to hide a lot of swelling and the bandage is to apply some make up powder. I actually have a make up stick which I have had for years. For a guy this feels a bit of strange thing to buy or carry, but a few dabs of a this on top and you can't even see it yourself close up in the mirror. The secret is to take a new Q-tip and work the end between your finger and thumb to loosen the cotton so it is more fluffy. Then dip it in the powder and roll it gently across the liquid bandage and surrounding area where necessary. A cheap small compact of powder is fine for this and I found a darker color was better as most are too light and the attempted disguise looks worse than no disguise.

Using the liquid bandage and lysine cream together

The secret is to use a small amount of liquid bandage to only cover the small area where the blister will break. If you do this you can then apply lysine cream around the small liquid bandage patch to help treat any swelling and further discourage a breakout. Be aware that gravity will play its part, so don't put too much cream above the patch. Try doing the sides first with a Q tip, then below and then with less left on the Q tip you can go above the patch. Again this is best if you are not going out and then you can leave the cream to be absorbed into the skin. The patch will be fine with a certain amount of cream as it is waterproof, but if it is completely covered so it can't itself breath it may work its way off.

Sometimes you may just need to cover the whole spot area with the liquid bandage and not bother with lysine cream at first. You may be late on it and it has burst. You might want to be sure you have it all covered. A cold sore can swell up so much, that you become worried it will bust from the side. One disadvantage with preventing the cold sore from bursting is that it might swell up a lot more than it would have if it had been allowed to burst. But if you used the ice effectively first, this should not happen. If it has, it can also be quite painful with the pressure of the swelling. It is a trade off. It looks worse on the first day, but you won't get the scab which lasts for many days. With this route, after a day or two you will be close to back to normal.

You may find yourself feeling that cold sore has burst below the liquid bandage. It is shinny anyway and it can be hard to tell. If you are not sure, try holding a piece of tissue across it again and see if any drops of liquid show on the tissue. Often they won't show up and you are just being paranoid. One tell-tale sign that you haven't managed to prevent the cold sore breaking is that the liquid bandage goes an orangey yellow, showing some mild infection showing through.

How long should you leave the liquid bandage on? Ideally until the swelling goes down. It is tempting to want to take it off and see how things are, but I have learned that the ideal is to leave that first application on for at least 12 hours. Ideally it best left on for a day, maybe even two. Sometimes it does get a bit crusty round the edges when the swelling has gone down. You can always apply a bit more on top to ensure the center of the spot is properly covered.

Removing the liquid bandage

The first application of liquid bandage should stay on until you try and remove it. It bonds quite strongly to the skin. If it has come lose around the surfaces, this is normally because the swelling has gone down. That's a good sign. Don't try and peel it off. There is a very good chance you will take skin with it and then open the wound and then scab and possibly scar.

There are three ways to remove the liquid bandage. The first is, as the manufacturers recommend, to apply more liquid bandage which will momentarily liquefy the old dried bandage allowing you to remove it. My preferred method is to cover it with lysine cream and allow it to soften for say 10 to 20 minutes and then use a Q tip to dislodge it. If it is not coming off very easily, apply more cream and let is soak longer. It should not be a struggle to get it off. The third method is to have a shower with it on, which is the best way to keep the sore area protected, and then use either of the first two methods to remove it.

How do you know when it is safe to remove the liquid bandage? If you managed to control the scale of a potential breakout with lysine tablets, then you may not even need to cover the area. You may only need a day and if you are not sure a second day. If, when you remove it, you find the skin is punctured apply a new liquid bandage again for another day or two and go through the same removal process again. Because it is transparent, you can normally tell when it has done its job and is safe to be removed.

If you feel uncomfortable using liquid bandage on your face, that's completely understandable. Simply use the patches instead, but I find they are not as good.

Dealing with redness

Once you have removed the liquid bandage you will probably still have some redness or a slightly raised area. You are effectively much where you would have been down the line if you had allowed a scab to form and fall off in several days time. You can continue to use lysine cream but switching to something for scarred skin, such as Bio Oil can also be effective. The skin might not be quite as robust as if it had healed under a scab and may take another day or so to tighten and fully recover.

If you have a scab forming

With the instructions above, you should avoid getting a scab all together. The scab is the most visible aspect to other people that you have a cold sore. It lengthens the time you have one and it is very hard to disguise. You may have been unlucky and ended up with a scab because you haven't caught things in time. Maybe you haven't yet managed to try out the method above. You may have rubbed the area in bed or by accident with a towel, putting on a top, damaged it swimming, or got sunburnt.

Scabs can take ages to heal if they are too disrupted. They can itch and be hard to leave alone and they can get infected. These are other good reasons for working to avoid getting one. If you have a scab it is best to let it run its coarse and fall off on its own accord as tempting as it is to peel it off. If you do try and remove it early, the area may be scared permanently.

Healing - Keep the scab moist

There are varying schools of thought on this, but nearly all the research suggests that healing will be faster if you keep the scab moist. You can do this with antiseptic cream. I have found that Quantum Health Lip Clear lysine cream had the right consistency when applied sparingly to a scab. Avoid the scab being so wet that it breaks up all the time only to reform again. One big disadvantage of keeping the scab moist is that this makes it hard to disguise with make up.

One problem with keeping the scab moist is that it can gunk up a bit. You may notice this especially after getting it wet in the shower when the scab gets a white consistency to it. The secret is not to use too much cream, but enough to keep it moist. If you do need to reduce the gunk, loosen the end of a q-tip (cotton bud) with your finger in order to fluff it up. Then roll the end very gently over the scab. You may need to do this a few times with new q-tips. Be careful not to lift the scab itself, this is just to remove the residue on it. After showering it can pay to let the area dry for a while first, before applying a small amount of cream to moisten it again.

Once the scab does fall off, you may have some redness where the skin is not fully recovered. Again Bio Oil is good to apply to the area until there are no signs of any lasting scaring. I also use the same Lip Clear Lysine cream by Quantum Health to help with healing.

Be careful with exposure to direct sunlight, which inhibits scars healing properly, or protect the area with sunscreen or SPF lip balm until it is fully healed.

Finally, if the area is itchy, this is a sure sign that the healing process is underway. Avoid any temptation to touch.

Hygiene

We have touched on this under showering, but it really is worth stressing that if you have a breakout the virus is highly contagious. There is a very high risk of passing it to other parts of your body, or other people or both. A few dos and don'ts:

- Wash your hands, and again. It is worth washing your hands before and after going to the toilet. This can feel a little embarrassing in a public toilet, but that's still better than giving yourself genital herpes for life. Hand sanitizer is also a useful thing to carry
- Don't share towels and indeed be careful when using your own. A clean towel each day during a breakout is wise
- Have a separate hand towel from your bath towel
- Don't share cups and glasses, spoons, forks, don't double dip into dips with things that have been in your mouth
- Don't engage in oral sex and be careful with any physical contact with others and yourself
- Learn to air kiss. Cheek to cheek don't touch your lips to someone's face
- Don't kiss children, especially babies. They are more susceptible to the virus than adults
- Keep your hands away from your mouth. Hard if you are a nail biter...like me
- Abstain from flossing your teeth during an outbreak
- Don't rub your eyes (I have read there is a risk of blindness) or nose. These entrances to your body are also susceptible to cold sores

Foods that aid healing

Once you have a cold sore well underway you are entering healing mode already. You will normally feel an itching in the cold sore area. With the technique above this can be as early as day two or three. Lysine will have an impact before and at the first signs of an outbreak, but focusing on which foods will most help healing once you have a scab is key. A general rule is that foods that are red, orange or yellow in color aid healing the most. The short list for foods that aid healing are:

- protein - meat, beans, eggs, dairy - especially yoghurt
- vitamin C - citrus fruits and juices, berries, tomatoes, peppers, cruciferous vegetables
- vitamin A - dark green leafy vegetables, carrots, cantaloupe
- Zinc - red meat, seafood - especially oysters

Turmeric is another food which may have significant benefits for healing and general health with a growing body of evidence that it may be the most effective natural supplement in existence. It is the spice that gives curry its yellow color and has been used in India as a spice and medicinal herb for over a thousand years. It is readily available in supplement form which might be worth considering during times of vulnerability and recovery.

The three dietary phases with cold sores

I have come to find there are there are three main phases with diet when it comes to cold sores:

1. High Nutrition Diet - keeping immunity high and reducing vulnerability
2. High Lysine Diet - when increased vulnerability or signs of an outbreak
3. High Healing Diet - to speed up recovery after increasing lysine

The foods to remember that are good for all three of these phases are:

- yoghurt - good probiotic for immunity, high in lysine and good for healing
- beets (beetroot) - good nutrition, high in lysine, good for healing
- cheese - lower nutrition, high in lysine, protein for healing
- mango - low pesticides, high in lysine, good for healing
- apple - medium nutrition, high in lysine, medium healing
- avocado - good nutrition, good for lysine, medium healing

- salmon - medium nutrition, good for lysine, good for healing
- tomato - good nutrition, good for lysine, good for healing
- green leaf vegetables - very high nutrition, medium lysine, good for healing
- eggs - medium nutrition, medium lysine, good for healing
- cruciferous vegetables - very high nutrition, medium lysine, good for healing
- carrots - very high nutrition, medium lysine, good for healing
- cantaloupe - very high nutrition, medium lysine, good for healing
- berries - good nutrition, medium lysine, good for healing

There are many other foods with excellent health properties too such as turmeric and ginger, but the foods listed above are some every day foods that are good for you at any time as a cold sore sufferer. Many foods will have a downside for at least one of these phases and this is especially true when it comes to lysine. Garlic, is great for nutrition for example but has an arginine to lysine ration or 2.5 to 1. So, at times of vulnerability that's a consideration.

Think about which of these foods you can really get into. I love dried mango for example. It is not quite as good as the fresh fruit, but it's an easy snack I know I will actually eat. It is easy to eat an apple a day as the infamous adage suggests. A carrot from the fridge is an easy snack. Carrots are also one of the easiest things to juice. Many nutritionists suggest juicing vegetables and eating fruit as most fruit juices are high in sugar. You can drink a big glass of orange juice, but try eating the same amount of fruit.

For many people, green vegetables are not so exciting but we all need to eat more of them. Order an extra portion of vegetables when you are out for dinner. Chose the fish on the menu instead of that big steak and add the vegetables. Get into making vegetable soups. Avocado cut in half with some olive oil and black pepper is delicious. Cheese and tomato is a great combo.

Start your day with yogurt and berries. I add chia or flax seeds, which are one of the highest sources of protein. But remember seeds are high in lysine, so lay of the seeds at times of vulnerability.

Once you begin to understand your times of vulnerability eating well to strengthen your immunity becomes habit. I have found a soup maker is great for creating soups for all three phases – prevention through high nutrition and immunity – i.e. greens, treatment through high lysine balance – i.e. beets, healing through color – i.e. carrots and peppers in soup.

Building a cold sore first aid kit

We have already seen the key things you need from a pharmacy in the event of a cold sore outbreak. Life gets a lot better if you are able to deal with a cold sore any time, any place. I generally have a few kits. I have a full kit at home with everything I might need in my bathroom cabinet. This can also be used to replenish my mobile kits. I have the essentials in my travel wash bag and another set in my laptop bag, which I am likely to have on a plane or at a conference or meeting. For women, a handbag is an obvious place to have what you need. You may not keep a kit as such, just the essential things floating around the bottom of a bag. I like to have a small plastic zip bag with these things in, so that I know for sure I have them. I feel more confident knowing I have what I need and will be less stressed if I get an outbreak coming. It is a bit like the feeling that it doesn't rain when you carry an umbrella.

Full kit - bathroom cabinet at home

- Lysine tablets - in a couple of jars
- Liquid bandage - a couple of bottles
- Q tips (cotton buds) - a full pack
- Zovirax – a couple of small tubes
- Lysine cream - Lip Clear Lysine + by Quantum Health is my favorite
- SPF Lip Balm - Herpicin HL 30 is my favorite
- Alcohol swabs for cleaning

- Bio Oil for healing
- Electric razor for shaving, which goes in my wash bag when I travel
- Also making sure the freezer is stocked up with ice/frozen tubs

Mobile kits - travel wash bag, hand bag, laptop bag

- Lysine tablets - I keep this in small pill boxes
- Liquid bandage - a small bottle
- Q tips (cotton buds) - just several loose
- Lysine and Zovirax creams
- SPF Lip Balm

There are key items that I have hidden in the car, boat and various jacket pockets (i.e. sailing or skiing) are:

- Lysine/Zovirax cream - Lip Clear Lysine + by Quantum Health is my favorite
- SPF Lip Balm - Herpicin HL 30 is my favorite

I actually buy these items when I see them in the pharmacy and have several of them dotted around so I can always find them for protection as a precaution. Having nothing to hand in the case of potentially risky conditions or the early signs of an outbreak is your worst nightmare.

8.   Stopping cold sores for good - Conclusion

This book is not promoting some miracle cure. All cold sore sufferers wish there was one. It is designed to help you understand how to avoid getting cold sores and how to manage them better. I have explained what I have found works for me and perhaps more importantly what doesn't. You may find in your own case that some things work better than others, but hopefully the previous chapters will get you to the answers more quickly.

The three main objectives you should strive for to stop getting cold sores are:

1. Avoid the conditions that lead to an outbreak - know your vulnerability
2. If you do enter a time of vulnerability - take preventative action
3. Head a cold sore off at the early stages - prevent it breaking out

In avoiding the conditions that lead to an outbreak, it is important that you build an understanding over time of what your vulnerabilities are. The Perfect Storm chapter outlines a set of scenarios. Is one of these your own perfect storm? Chapter 5 focuses on knowing your vulnerability and it is worth recording any of the conditions outlined there in the run up to getting a cold sore. Knowledge is everything and building a true understanding of why you get cold sores in the first place will help you to minimize getting them going forward.

When I first started getting cold sores, I would get several a year. At times it seemed, I had no sooner got rid of one and then I would get another one. It could literally be a few weeks between outbreaks. If this is happening to you, it is almost certainly that your immune system is constantly low. Your diet and your lysine/Arginine balance will need a serious review.

Now I get one or two a year which I consistently manage to reverse from actually breaking out. For me these are nearly always in the fall when the weather turns and I myself feel under the weather. I have learned to spot the signs of feeling tired around this time. Here I take some preventative measures by getting lots of sleep, avoiding going out in the cold and increasing my lysine/arginine balance through diet and tablets. At these times, I don't touch nuts and eat more cheese. Some winters, I now manage to avoid getting a cold sore altogether. Since writing the first edition of this book, I have had whole years of not getting a cold sore at all without any intervention. I put this down to better understanding of my health and vulnerability.

In the pervious chapter we look at swinging into action to head off a cold sore at the early stages. Before I discovered this technique of stopping a cold sore fully developing, it was a good two weeks before I felt I could confidently go out again. The cold sore would burst after a couple of days and I would have the trials and tribulations of dealing with a messy scab that could take well over a week to heal.

Using the combination of ice and lysine tablets my cold sores are at best reversed in a day or at worst swell up but back under control in two days. I might cancel engagements for a day or two to be sure I am getting rest and dealing with it properly. But I find a feel absolutely confident about accepting an invitation to go out in two or three nights time. Previously I couldn't be confident when a cold sore would be gone and would worry about a date or meeting friends. I felt I was becoming a bit of a hermit living in fear of the next outbreak. Just getting your confidence back will be a big help in itself.

Improving your diet, sleeping well, getting more exercise and keeping warmer in winter should all have added health benefits in improving your immune system the major reason why you get cold sore outbreaks.

In this book I have shared my own voyage of discovery in dealing with cold sores over many years. It is the book I would have liked to have had when I first started dealing with them myself. I really hope it helps you, saves you time and a lot of anguish going forward.

Please persevere with it and be patient. It may take you a few outbreaks to master the practical techniques I have explained. I strongly recommend that each time you get a cold sore coming, you refer to this book to understand what triggered it to help you avoid it next time. Read and re-

read it when you get a cold sore so you can reduce the impact each time and learn to reverse them as I have done.

Please recommend this book to anyone you know who suffers from cold sores and even when you see someone with one. If we can stop outbreaks among the population, we may ultimately start to reduce this virulent medical problem.

I never thought I would say this, but living with cold sores is not that bad. Once you master how to handle them, life really does get better. The techniques outlined in this book have really worked for me. Hopefully they will work for you too!

Finally - Remember to eat well, sleep well, exercise and keep warm in winter. Good luck.

Please, please review my book. The more people we help the better.

I welcome any feedback at: coldsorebook@gmail.com

Appendix A - Lysine v Arginine Tables

The table below ranks the ratio of Lysine to Arginine in common foods

Food	Ratio Lys/Arg	Food	Ratio Lys/Arg	Food	Ratio Lys/Arg
Margarine	3.00	Chicken	1.41	Carrots	0.92
Plain Yogurt	2.98	Pineapple	1.39	Watercress	0.86
Swiss Cheese	2.79	Pork	1.37	Swiss chard	0.86
Edam Cheese	2.76	Potato	1.36	Eggplant	0.84
American Cheese Spread	2.76	Celery	1.33	Peas	0.74
Whey, dry, sweet	2.75	Beef steak	1.32	Brussels sprouts	0.73
Blue Cheese	2.60	Ham, boneless	1.31	Orange	0.73
Papaya	2.53	Turkey	1.29	Mushrooms	0.67
Brie Cheese	2.52	Pork sausage	1.29	Cucumber	0.61
Parmesan Cheese	2.51	Peach	1.25	Wheat, shredded	0.59
Beets	2.40	Ground beef, lean	1.24	Wheat flakes	0.59
Mozzarella Cheese	2.37	Green beans	1.21	Bran flakes	0.56
Processed American Cheese	2.37	Pork Bacon	1.21	Cashews	0.52
Butter	2.25	Salami, hard	1.20	Pumpkin seeds	0.45
Cheddar Cheese	2.20	Lettuce	1.16	Garlic	0.42
Ice Cream	2.19	Cauliflower	1.13	Blackberries	0.35
Whole Milk	2.19	Spinach	1.09	Blueberries	0.35
Mango	2.18	Kale	1.07	Onions	0.34
Apricot	2.15	Whole Egg	1.06	Grapes	0.31
Apple	2.13	Corn	1.05	Peanut butter	0.29
Pear	1.92	Sweet potato	1.05	Peanuts	0.29
Apricot, dried	1.82	Banana	1.02	Coconut, shredded	0.27
Avocado	1.59	Asparagus	1.01	Almonds	0.27
Salmon	1.55	Oat flakes	1.01	Pecans	0.27
Whitefish	1.54	Mayonnaise	1.00	Sesame seeds	0.25
Tuna, in water	1.53	Leeks	1.00	Brazil nuts	0.23
Cod	1.53	Shrimp	0.99	Pine nuts	0.19
Sardines, in oil, drained	1.53	Crab	0.99	Orange juice	0.19
Halibut	1.53	Broccoli	0.97	Walnuts	0.19
Tomato	1.52	Strawberries	0.95	Hazelnuts	0.19

This table below ranks the amount of Lysine in mg per 100g (3.5oz - about a handful) in common foods. For liquids, 100g or water is 100ml. Cheese scores very highly, while you would need to eat a lot of mango or apple (which have high lysine-arginine ratios) to get similar quantities of lysine.

Food	Lys mg/100g	Food	Lys mg/100g	Food	Lys mg/100g
Parmesan Cheese	3,346	Pork sausage	900	Lettuce	104
Tuna, in water	2,715	Sesame seeds	827	Swiss chard	100
Edam Cheese	2,693	Whole Egg	820	Apricot	90
Swiss Cheese	2,618	Mayonnaise	757	Green beans	88
Mozzarella Cheese	2,496	Almonds	666	Sweet potato	81
Sardines, in oil, drained	2,258	Pork Bacon	639	Leeks	78
Processed American Cheese	2,225	Brazil nuts	541	Avocado	69
Cheddar Cheese	2,100	Walnuts	466	Mushrooms	69
Turkey	1,967	Bran flakes	377	Margarine	64
Chicken	1,966	Hazelnuts	340	Butter	64
Halibut	1,906	Wheat, shredded	335	Onions	56
Blue Cheese	1,879	Peas	317	Beets	53
Brie Cheese	1,875	Plain Yogurt	311	Eggplant	51
Salmon	1,824	Wheat flakes	306	Carrots	40
Salami, hard	1,820	Pecans	292	Orange	34
Pumpkin seeds	1,807	Ice Cream	286	Tomato	33
Shrimp	1,765	Garlic	267	Banana	31
Whitefish	1,753	Whole Milk	261	Mango	28
Pork	1,663	Apricot, dried	254	Celery	27
Cod	1,635	Kale	197	Pineapple	25
Beef steak	1,612	Spinach	178	Strawberries	25
Crab	1,588	Watercress	165	Cucumber	21
American Cheese Spread	1,525	Cashews	154	Peach	17
Ham, boneless	1,487	Brussels sprouts	148	Papaya	17
Ground beef, lean	1,478	Coconut, shredded	148	Grapes	15
Oat flakes	1,215	Asparagus	145	Pear	13
Peanut butter	1,173	Broccoli	141	Blackberries	12
Whey, dry, sweet	1,027	Corn	136	Blueberries	12
Peanuts	1,007	Potato	127	Apple	11
Pine nuts	914	Cauliflower	108	Orange juice	9

This table ranks the amount of Arginine in mg per 100g (3.5oz - about a handful) in common foods. For liquids, 100g or water is 100ml. Nuts and seeds score very highly here and are therefore bad for cold sores. Note, you would need to eat a lot of berries (which low lysine-arginine ratios) to be taking in dangerous levels of arginine.

Food	Arg mg/100g	Food	Arg mg/100g	Food	Arg mg/100g
Pine nuts	4,750	Swiss Cheese	939	Mushrooms	103
Peanut butter	4,087	Processed American Cheese	939	Cauliflower	96
Pumpkin seeds	3,979	Whole Egg	776	Potato	93
Peanuts	3,507	Mayonnaise	757	Lettuce	89
Sesame seeds	3,327	Brie Cheese	743	Leeks	78
Walnuts	2,520	Blue Cheese	721	Sweet potato	77
Almonds	2,493	Pork sausage	700	Green beans	73
Brazil nuts	2,393	Bran flakes	668	Eggplant	61
Hazelnuts	1,837	Garlic	633	Grapes	49
Shrimp	1,776	Wheat, shredded	564	Orange	47
Tuna, in water	1,770	American Cheese Spread	554	Orange juice	47
Crab	1,600	Coconut, shredded	546	Avocado	44
Turkey	1,522	Pork Bacon	529	Carrots	44
Salami, hard	1,520	Wheat flakes	518	Apricot	42
Sardines, in oil, drained	1,475	Peas	428	Cucumber	35
Chicken	1,398	Whey, dry, sweet	373	Blackberries	34
Parmesan Cheese	1,332	Cashews	294	Blueberries	34
Halibut	1,247	Brussels sprouts	202	Banana	31
Beef steak	1,222	Watercress	192	Butter	28
Pork	1,218	Kale	184	Strawberries	26
Oat flakes	1,206	Onions	164	Beets	22
Ground beef, lean	1,195	Spinach	164	Tomato	22
Salmon	1,176	Broccoli	145	Margarine	21
Whitefish	1,142	Asparagus	143	Celery	20
Ham, boneless	1,139	Apricot, dried	140	Pineapple	18
Pecans	1,102	Ice Cream	131	Peach	14
Cod	1,066	Corn	130	Mango	13
Mozzarella Cheese	1,054	Whole Milk	119	Pear	7
Edam Cheese	975	Swiss chard	117	Papaya	7
Cheddar Cheese	954	Plain Yogurt	104	Apple	5

This last table ranks the portion size of food in grams you would need to eat to match a 500mg lysine tablet (100g = 3.5oz - about a handful) for common foods. For liquids, 100g or water is 100ml. Cheese scores very highly again with fish. You would need to eat a lot of fruit to get similar quantities of lysine. The foods marked with an asterisk * have over twice as much arginine. A handful of nuts gives a fair amount of lysine but much more arginine.

Food	Portion in g to 500mg Lysine	Food	Portion in g to 500mg Lysine	Food	Portion in g to 500mg Lysine
Parmesan Cheese	15	Pork sausage	56	Lettuce	483
Tuna, in water	18	Sesame seeds*	60	Swiss chard	500
Edam Cheese	19	Whole Egg	61	Apricot	553
Swiss Cheese	19	Mayonnaise	66	Green beans	567
Mozzarella Cheese	20	Almonds*	75	Sweet potato	619
Sardines, in oil, drained	22	Pork Bacon	78	Leeks	639
Processed American Cheese	22	Brazil nuts*	92	Avocado	720
Cheddar Cheese	24	Walnuts*	107	Mushrooms	729
Turkey	25	Bran flakes*	133	Margarine	783
Chicken	25	Hazelnuts*	147	Butter	783
Halibut	26	Wheat, shredded*	149	Onions*	889
Blue Cheese	27	Peas	158	Beets	944
Brie Cheese	27	Plain Yogurt	161	Eggplant	976
Salmon	27	Wheat flakes	163	Carrots	1,250
Salami, hard	27	Pecans*	171	Orange	1,452
Pumpkin seeds	28	Ice Cream	175	Tomato	1,500
Shrimp	28	Garlic*	188	Banana	1,591
Whitefish	29	Whole Milk	192	Mango	1,765
Pork	30	Apricot, dried	197	Celery	1,875
Cod	31	Kale	254	Pineapple	1,987
Beef steak	31	Spinach	281	Strawberries	2,014
Crab	31	Watercress	302	Cucumber	2,364
American Cheese Spread	33	Cashews	325	Peach	2,875
Ham, boneless	34	Brussels sprouts	338	Papaya	2,987
Ground beef, lean	34	Coconut, shredded*	339	Grapes*	3,333
Oat flakes	41	Asparagus	345	Pear	3,913
Peanut butter*	43	Broccoli	355	Blackberries*	4,265
Whey, dry, sweet	49	Corn	367	Blueberries*	4,265
Peanuts*	50	Potato	395	Apple	4,412
Pine nuts*	55	Cauliflower	463	Orange juice*	5,636